THE LOW-OXALATE
FOOD LIST

BY MORGAN F. WHITTAKER

LEGAL & DISCLAIMER

The information contained in this book is not designed to replace or take the place of any form of medicine or professional medical advice. The information in this book has been provided for educational and entertainment purposes only.

You need to consult a professional medical practitioner in order to ensure you are both healthy enough and able to make use of this information. Always consult your professional medical practitioner before undertaking any new dietary regime, and particularly after reading this book.

The information contained in this book has been compiled from sources deemed reliable, and it is accurate to the best of the Author's knowledge; however, the Author cannot guarantee its accuracy and validity and cannot be held liable for any errors or omissions.

You must consult your doctor or get professional medical advice before using any suggested information in this book.

Contents

Introduction

Congratulations on choosing this book. It was written out of frustration with the conflicting and confusing information about food intolerances and oxalate issues.

Essentially, one list will tell you something is low oxalate, and another high oxalate.

The National Library of Medicine's research paper details these issues. Their conclusion was this;

"Wide variations exist in the reported oxalate content of foods across several Web-based sources and smartphone applications, several of which are substantial and can have a sizable impact on the construction of a low oxalate diet. As dietary counseling has proven benefits, patients and caregivers should be aware of the heterogeneity that exists in the reported oxalate content of foods."

This book gathers the world's best and most trusted oxalate lists and guides and compiles the information into one easy-to-consult guide. Trust this process; it's been quite the journey.

Even during the compilation of this guide, it was noticed that many of the top lists massively disagree on oxalate content in food.

As is now understood, that's the nature of oxalate content and issues. Everybody reacts differently, and foods even show up differently depending on the growing process, variety, season, soil conditions, time of harvest, and many other factors (Pitchaporn Wanyo, Kannika Huaisan & Tossaporn Chamsai).

That's why this list was created. It is believed to be the most comprehensive out there, and where there is debate, deference has been given to many of these top sources. With all that said, there will be areas you disagree on, and that is why a) approach any new food with caution, and b) always consult your medical practitioner before making any dietary changes.

This list will never be definitive, and will continue to be refined as more information becomes available. But it means you must approach every food cautiously.

There will be no rehashing of the reasons behind your oxalate issues. You've almost certainly done your research on it, and that's why you are here, for the most comprehensive low-oxalate food list available.

If you have oxalate issues, no matter what kind, use this book to avoid foods that are high in oxalates. These include major culprits like spinach and rhubarb, but also lesser-known culprits like almonds. Almonds are in themselves individually fairly low in oxalate but there is an issue with portion control - remember what was previously about portion-size? One or two almonds - fine. The whole packet = lots of oxalates.

So you'll learn all about what to avoid from this book, and you might start to feel a lot better from your oxalate issues.

It's also important to point out that not everybody needs to avoid oxalates. As the website Healthline notes;

Some proponents of low-oxalate diets say people are better off not consuming foods rich in oxalates, since they may have negative health effects. However, it's not that simple. Many of these are healthy foods that contain important antioxidants, fiber and other nutrients. Therefore, it's not a good idea for most people to completely stop eating high-oxalate foods.

All of which means you should consult with your practitioner to determine the correct course for you. Please keep in mind that materials and resources like this book are no substitute for medical advice and not intended as such.

Without further ado, let's get straight on to the food list.

How to use this food list

This book works like a dictionary. Look for a food, drink or ingredient alphabetically or on search.

Once you find what you are looking for, it is scored between 1 and 5 for oxalate levels based on careful analysis of the world's best sources (listed below) for oxalate content.

Some online titles detail either cup size, serving size or precise amount of mg of oxalates per 100 g. That can be really useful, but most of us get hungry, and that means one person's servings might be be three of somebody else's.

So things are more straightforward in this book. In consultation with all the major sites, lists and experts, each food gets a score. The higher the score, the better it is for your low oxalate diet.

- 5 is best (indicates good choice for a low-oxalate diet as per sources)
- 1 is worst (indicates poor choice for a low-oxalate diet as per sources)

So on a low-oxalate diet, 5 is best and 1 is worst. You would look to be initially consuming more 5 foods and cutting out 1 foods. As time goes on, with the help of a skilled practitioner, you would look to address the root cause of your oxalate issues and perhaps reintroducing foods as possible to get a varied and nutritious diet.

A scoring system has been used because many food lists only group foods into 'high' or 'low' oxalate (or 'bad' and 'good'. It was felt there is considerably more nuance to food intolerances, allergies and analysis. Respected sites can disagree on major foods so that is reflected that in this book.

You'll also find 'at-a-glance' lists of high and low oxalate foods to help you on your journey.

At this point; a disclaimer. The aim is to heal from oxalate issues, and live a healthy, balanced life in every aspect. This book has been a labour of love, but it has been a challenge to put together as the major lists disagree so often about oxalate content. You must consult your doctor or get professional medical advice before using any suggested information in this book. This is a guide, not a definitive list as everybody is individual.

Keep this book close by when you cook or eat out, and dip in and out whenever you need to check if something is low oxalate.

Sources

These excellent sources are very highly recommended in your further research on oxalates. As far as possible these sites and many more (plus personal experience) have been consulted in the research into this food list.

The major sites vary considerably which is the reason for the book.

This entire book comes with the caveat that absolutely everybody reacts differently to certain foods, and therefore oxalate food lists are important but you should always consult your practitioner and do further reading.

Please do click on these top oxalate diet sites for further reading. All of them are highly recommended. They are some of the best sources out there - even if they do disagree with each other!

- The University of Chicago - How To Eat A Low Oxalate Diet https://kidneystones.uchicago.edu/how-to-eat-a-low-oxalate-diet/

- Harvard T.H. Chan School of Public Health https://regepi.bwh.harvard.edu/health/Oxalate/files

- Harvard T.H. Chan School of Public Health Food List https://regepi.bwh.harvard.edu/health/Oxalate/files/Oxalate%20Content%20of%20Foods.xls

- National Library of Medicine - Oxalate content of food: a tangled web https://pubmed.ncbi.nlm.nih.gov/25168533/

- University of Virginia - Digestive Health Center https://med.virginia.edu/ginutrition/wp-content/uploads/sites/199/2014/04/Oxalate-Foods-02.17.pdf

- Pitchaporn Wanyo, Kannika Huaisan & Tossaporn Chamsai - Oxalate contents of Thai rice paddy herbs (*L. aromatica* and *L. geoffrayi*) are affected by drying method and changes after cooking https://link.springer.com/article/10.1007/s42452-020-2703-6

- Urinary Stones Info - The Oxalate Content Of Food https://www.urinarystones.info/resources/Docs/Oxalate-content-of-food-2008.pdf

- Low Oxalate Info Website http://lowoxalateinfo.com/

- Winchester Hospital Low-Oxalate Diet Health Library https://www.winchesterhospital.org/health-library/article?id=196214

- Low-Oxalate Diet - Mark O'Brien MD (adapted from University of Pittsburgh Medical Center https://www.markobrienmd.com/OxalateDiet.pdf

- University of Michigan Health - Foods High in Oxalate https://www.uofmhealth.org/health-library/aa166321

The Food List

- 5 is best (indicates good for a low-oxalate diet as per sources above)
- 1 is worst (indicates poor choice for low-oxalate diet as per sources above)

Acerola: 4

Acerola contains a lot of vitamin C. In large doses, it might cause kidney stones in some people.

Agave syrup: 2

One of those very confusing ingredients that is listed as low oxalate on many lists, but agave itself is listed as very high on many other lists. This is why this book was written, and ultimately, if you want to eat agave on a low-oxalate diet, proceed with great caution as there is some debate about the oxalate content.

Alcohol: 4

Beer is thought to be low-oxalate. Red wine and white wine are thought to be very low, and liquor extremely low.

So alcohol actually gets quite a good score in the list. With of course, the usual caveats about other health-related issues linked to alcohol. Alcohol might often be low oxalate, but it might also not be good for your health.

Algae: 4

Related to Algae, phycocyanin in spirulina (a blue green algae) can protect cells from oxalates. This is according to a research article published by the National Institute of Health.

Almond: 1

With almonds, and all nuts, there is an issue with portion control - remember what was said previously about portion-size?

One or two almonds will probably be okay for you However, the whole packet = lots of oxalates. Almonds can very quickly cause oxalate issues.

Some say all nuts should be avoided on a Low-Oxalate diet. Almonds and Brazil nuts are thought to be particularly high.

According to the University of Chicago, almonds contain 122mg per serving.

Anchovies: 4

Low in oxalates, but thought to be high in purines, which also cause kidney stones – uric ones, not calcium oxalate, which are the most common kind.

Apple: 5

Thought to be low oxalate.

Apple cider vinegar: 5

Low oxalate. The website Healthline notes an additional benefit.

Some people recommend using ACV as a natural way to treat kidney stones. The acetic acid found in ACV is thought to soften, break down, and dissolve kidney stones. The kidney stones can be reduced in size so that you're able to easily pass them in your urine.

Apricot: 5

Low oxalate, just 5–9 mg per 100 g (Source: University of Chicago).

Artichokes: 2

According to the University of Chicago, oxalate content of artichokes is moderate at 5 mg per one small bud.

Artificial sweeteners: 3

Most sweeteners are in the category of "very low" with 0.1 - 2.9 mg of oxalates per 100 g according to the Urology Care Foundation. You are still urged you to avoid artificial sweeteners for other, well-documented health reasons. Unfortunately, some natural sweeteners (which are often a better option) are higher in oxalates.

Asparagus: 3

Moderate in oxalates, 5 mg per 100 g (University of Chicago). According to the Oxalosis and Hyperoxaluria Foundation, asparagus contains 2 to 10 mg of oxalate in a one-half-cup serving which is also thought to be a moderate source.

Aubergine: 1

Also called Eggplant. The Winchester Hospital lists eggplant in their High Oxalate, Foods To Avoid list. The PainSpy site lists Eggplant as very high. Some disagreement over oxalate content but they've been listed as high.

Avocado: 1

Very high in oxalates, 19 mg per 100 g (The University of Chicago).

Bamboo shoots: 1

Thought to be very high in oxalate content.

Banana: 4

Low oxalate, just 5–9 mg per 100 g (University of Chicago).

Barley: 4

3.0 - 4.9 mg per 100 g, low oxalate (source: Open Nutrition Journal).

Barley malt, malt: 1

See malt.

Basil: 4

Not a massive amount of information out there, but UPMC lists as low-oxalate. Basil pesto with olive oil and a few almonds is an enjoyable recipe!

Beans: 1

Beans are generally high in oxalates. Kidney beans could be a better option with about 15 mg per half a cup, but beans generally = oxalates (Source: North Dakota State University).

Beef: 5

Meats are normally safe to eat on a low-oxalate diet. Remember, eating large portions of meat is thought to potentially increase the risk of kidney stones.

Organic meat is preferable to avoid fertilisers and pesticides. This is not oxalate-related, but for associated general health.

Beer: 4

Comments: See alcohol.

Beetroot: 1

Also known as Beets. Very high in oxalates - one of the highest foods around. The website Healthline notes; Levels of oxalates are much higher in the leaves than the root itself, but the root is nevertheless considered high in oxalates.

Bell pepper (hot): 1

Chili pepper is often categorized as high, 10.0-14.9 mg (source: Harvard).

Bell pepper (sweet): 3

Green pepper is thought to be moderate in oxalates, but it can be very high in pesticide residue. Best to buy organic.

Bison: 5

Most meats are low in oxalates. It would be great to eat more bison but it's hard to find in many parts of the world. It's generally a good alternative to beef with less saturated fat although in the research for this book there wasn't much available information on oxalates. It is likely low oxalate but as always test carefully. Remember, eating large portions of meat is thought to potentially increase the risk of kidney stones.

Bivalves (mussels, oyster, clams, scallops): 5

Generally thought to be low oxalate. (Who knew these seafoods were called bivalves?)

Black caraway: 1

According to research, extensive amounts of total oxalate (201-4014 mg/100 g D.W.) were found in daily common herbs such as caraway seed, green cardamom, cinnamon, coriander seeds, cumin, curry powder, ginger, and turmeric powder (source: The Canadian Center of Science and Education). Depends on the quantities used.

Blackberry: 3

Blueberries and blackberries have just 4 mg per cup (source: North Dakota State University). Also rich in antioxidants.

Blackcurrants: 2

Moderate in oxalates, should be limited.

Blue cheeses: 2

Dairy is free of oxalate. It's also high in calcium, so it is a good choice, although cheese can have other health implications. What about dressings? Blue cheese dressing has less than 5 mg of oxalates per 100 g (source: Urinary Stones - The Oxalate Content Of Food).

Blue fenugreek: 1

Very high; total oxalate of blue fenugreek powder amounted to 1246 mg/100 g. (source: Scientific Electronic Library Online of Brazil)

Blueberries: 3

Blueberries and blackberries have 4 mg per cup (source: a publication by North Dakota State University). Blueberries are also rich in antioxidants, which can help ward off cancer, heart disease, and other serious health conditions.

Bok choi: 5

Sometimes also written as *bok choy*. A lovely leafy green veg. Try sautéing or lightly roasting for 15 minutes.

Thought to be very low in oxalates - only around 1 mg per 100 g.

Borlotti beans: 1

See more general comments under *Beans.*

Bouillon: 1

Shop-bought stocks and bouillons can have a lot of different ingredients, so it's always worth checking closely. Very difficult to give a rating. Some of those ingredients; glutamate, yeast extract, spice (often high in oxalates)/ aroma/ flavor/ seasoning/ condiment, meat extracts, vegetables.

Boysenberry: 4

Low; 2-6 mg/100g (source: Journal of Food Composition and Analysis).

Brandy: 4

See "Alcohol"

Brazil nut: 1

Pine nuts, candle nuts, and Brazil nuts contain high levels of gastric soluble oxalate (492.0–556.8 mg/100 g). The intestinal soluble oxalate is the fraction that will be absorbed in the small intestine. (source: Journal of Food Composition and Analysis)

Bread: 2

Check the individual ingredients in this book. On close inspection of oxalate lists, corn and oatmeal bread are thought to be lower oxalate than wheat bread.

Also, the fermentation process and yeasting process is uncertain but you may well tolerate most breads.

Test with caution. You could even make your own with the ingredients that suit you.

That said, drugs.com notes these breads are low-to-medium oxalate foods to include in the diet:

White bread, cornbread, bagels, and white English muffins (medium oxalate)

In sum, breads can range from very high in oxalates (French toast with 13 mg per two slices) to low (oat bran, corn, and oatmeal bread with 4 mg per slice/piece).

Broad-leaved garlic: 5

All kinds of garlic, raw or cooked, are very low in oxalates (less than 5mg per 100 g).

Broad beans: 1

See comments on 'Beans'. Also known as Vicia Faba.

Broccoli: 3

According to the University of Chicago, half a cup of chopped broccoli has 6 mg of oxalates, which is moderate. The Pain Spy website considers broccoli to have 190mg of oxalates per 100g.

Brussels sprouts: 1

Thought to be high in oxalates. Avoid.

Buckwheat: 1

Buckwheat flour, whole-groat is listed as very high (15.0mg & up) (source: University of Chicago). In fact they list it as one of their highest oxalate foods, though they optimistically note:

Rhubarb and spinach are so high you just cannot eat them. Rice bran is something few will miss, the same for buckwheat groats.

Butter: 5

Thought to have little or no oxalates. That said, eating organic, grass-fed butter is important. It's easy to find. You should be able to find grass-fed, organic, and affordable butter in the supermarket or a specialized store.

Cabbage: 5

Cabbage is very versatile and cheap, and it's often affordable even when buying organic. It is thought to be very low in oxalates along with similar veggies like endive, cauliflower, and lettuce.

Cactus pear: 2

Proceed with caution. Studies suggest the oxalate content of cactus pears differs depending on whether they are raw or mature.

Cardamom: 1

Many spices are high in oxalates and cardamom appears to be one of the highest. This is from PubMed:

Spices, such as cinnamon, cloves, cardamom, garlic, ginger, cumin, coriander and turmeric are used all over the world as flavouring and colouring ingredients in Indian foods. Previous studies have shown that spices contain variable amounts of total oxalates but there are few reports of soluble oxalate contents. In this study, the total, soluble and insoluble oxalate contents of ten different spices commonly used in Indian cuisine were measured. Total oxalate content ranged from 194 (nutmeg) to 4,014 (green cardamom) mg/100 g DM, while the soluble oxalate contents ranged from 41 (nutmeg) to 3,977 (green cardamom) mg/100 g DM. Overall, the percentage of soluble oxalate content of the spices ranged from 4.7 to 99.1% of the total oxalate content which suggests that some spices present no risk to people liable to kidney stone formation, while other spices can supply significant amounts of soluble oxalates and therefore should be used in moderation.

Carrot: 2

Highish - one 100 g of carrot contains 15 mg of oxalates (source: St. Joseph's Healthcare Hamilton).

Cashew nut: 1

High. Nuts like walnuts and cashews are high but thought to have slightly lower levels of oxalates than almonds; about 30 mg per ounce (source: St. Joseph's Healthcare Hamilton).

Cassava: 2

Delicious as a flour but is it high in oxalates? This book has done lots of research on cassava as an ingredient and the lists tend to disagree and vary widely. So proceed with caution as some think cassava contains significant amounts of oxalates. As always, it may well be an individual thing, but cassava is one that can't get a high score.

Cauliflower: 5

Thought to be low in oxalates.

Celery: 1

High in oxalates, Listed as a 'Food to avoid' on the Unusual Ingredients website, and this verdict is borne out by many of the respected lists in sources table above.

Cep mushrooms: 4

See mushrooms.

Chamomile and chamomile tea: 5

Low, just 0.4-0.67 mg per cup (source: National Library of Medicine).

Champagne: 4

See alcohol.

Chard: 1

High in oxalate. One to put in your 'avoid' list.

Chard is known by a number of other popular names, including Swiss chard, silverbeet, leaf beet, Sicilian beet, Chilian beet, Roman kale, spinach beet or mangold.

Some experts believe just half a cup of steamed red swiss chard has even more oxalates than a half cup of steamed spinach.

All of which tells you chard, swiss chard, silverbeet, or whatever you want to call it, is on the avoid list on a low-oxalate diet.

Cheddar cheese: 5

See comments on cheeses below.

Cheese made from unpasteurized "raw" milk: 5

See comments on cheeses below.

Cheeses: 5

Most cheeses are low in oxalate or completely free of it. These include, among others;

- American Cheese
- Cheddar Cheese
- Low Fat Cheese Cottage Cheese
- Low Fat Cottage Cheese
- Cottage Cheese
- Cream Cheese
- Mozzarella Cheese

And other cheeses too.

This is because dairy is free of oxalate.

It's also high in calcium, so it is a good choice, although cheese can have other health implications which should be carefully considered.

Cherry: 4

Low oxalate, with different lists suggesting between 3-9 mg per 100 g

Chia, chia seeds: 1

Very high, 380 mg oxalate per quarter cup of chia seeds (Source: US National Library of Medicine). It should be noted that you may be consuming a much smaller amount than a quarter cup, but the oxalate levels will still be high.

Chicken: 5

Very low as long as it's organic and fresh.

Chickpeas: 3

Thought to be low to medium in oxalate. Sources tend to vary between 5-10mg per cup.

Chicory: 1

Some debate. Many consider it to be quite high in oxalates, with 21mg per 100g (Agriculture Handbook No. 8-11, Vegetables and Vegetable Products, 1984).

Chili pepper, red, fresh: 3

Hot chili peppers are thought to be moderate in oxalates. Red peppers are low.

Chives: 5

Low oxalate with less than 5mg per serving. (source: Urinary Stones website).

As emphasized throughout this book though, proceed with caution as the more you look into this area, the more debate there is.

The Agriculture Handbook No. 8-11, Vegetables and Vegetable Products, 1984 lists chives as high oxalate so proceed with caution.

The Heal With Food website notes;

Like parsley, chives are generally only used in small amounts in cooking. Therefore, chives are not likely to contribute much oxalic acid to your diet, despite the fact they are among the most concentrated dietary sources of oxalates. A 100-serving of chives is estimated to provide 1480 milligrams of oxalates.

Chocolate: 1

Chocolate is potentially high in oxalates. This from Science Direct:

As chocolate is considered as a high oxalate food (Williams and Wilson, 1990, Massey et al., 1993, Noonan and Savage, 1999, Mendonça et al., 2003), The Oxalosis & Hyperoxaluria Foundation (OHF, 2004) recommends that affected persons should avoid eating chocolate.

Note that white chocolate may be better tolerated on a low oxalate diet.

Cilantro: 4

Also called coriander. Low oxalate (source: Urinary Stones website). They (very specifically) note that this relates to 9 raw sprigs.

Cinnamon: 1

High oxalate as per a number of studies.

This from PubMed on spices:

Spices, such as cinnamon, cloves, cardamom, garlic, ginger, cumin, coriander and turmeric are used all over the world as flavouring and colouring ingredients in Indian foods. Previous studies have shown that spices contain variable amounts of total oxalates but there are few reports of soluble oxalate contents. In this study, the total, soluble and insoluble oxalate contents of ten different spices commonly used in Indian cuisine were measured. Total oxalate content ranged from 194 (nutmeg) to 4,014 (green cardamom) mg/100 g DM, while the soluble oxalate contents ranged from 41 (nutmeg) to 3,977 (green cardamom) mg/100 g DM. Overall, the percentage of soluble oxalate content of the spices ranged from 4.7 to 99.1% of the total oxalate content which suggests that some spices present no risk to people liable to kidney stone formation, while other spices can supply significant amounts of soluble oxalates and therefore should be used in moderation.

Citrus fruits: 3

Varies. For example, oranges are very high, lemons are low. Check individual foods.

Clover: 1

Very high, contains oxalic acid, which depletes the body of calcium and iron. Red clover is toxic.

Cloves: 1

Very high in oxalate. Thought to be one of the highest oxalate-containing spices.

Cocoa butter and cacao butter: 1

High oxalate. Note the below from PubMed:

Cocoa is a strong carrier of oxalic acid (average: 400 mg per 100 g). In three calcium oxalate stone formers clinical observation had been suggestive of excessive intake of cocoa products contributing to calculus formation.

Cocoa drinks, powder, etc: 1

High oxalate. Note the below from Heal With Food:

A 2011 study published in the Journal of Food Composition and Analysis found that the total oxalate content of cocoa powder can range from 650 to 783 milligrams per 100 grams on a dry matter basis (cocoa powder contains very little moisture which implies the values would be very similar on a wet weight basis).

Coconut and coconut derivatives: 5

Low in oxalates according to a number of sources.

Coffee: 5

Low oxalate. Thank goodness for that!

Coriander: 4

See cilantro.

Corn salad, lamb's lettuce: 5

See lettuce

Cornflakes: 5

There are a number of foods that might be well-tolerated in terms of oxalates but are not going to be particularly good for your overall health. Let's put cornflakes into that category. Online specialist The Kidney Dietitian notes;

Rice Chex, Rice Krispies, cornflakes and Cheerios are very low oxalate cereal choices.... Some cold cereals are very high in oxalate – be careful to avoid bran flakes (yes, that includes Raisin Bran), rice bran and shredded wheat. These all have more than 25 grams of oxalate per 100 g.

However, there are healthier breakfast options.

Elsewhere in the world of corn, the website Kidney Cop lists corn flour as low-oxalate and safe to consume.

Courgette: 5

Thought to have less than 2 mg of oxalate per serving.

Crab: 5

Low.

Cranberries and cranberry juice: 3

Opinion varies so proceed with caution. This is one food that has been updated in this version of the book as more relevant research is considered.

In particular we looked at this study suggesting high oxalate levels.

"The urinary oxalate levels in the volunteers significantly increased (P = 0.01) by an average of 43.4% while receiving cranberry tablets. The excretion of potential lithogenic ions calcium, phosphate, and sodium also increased. However, inhibitors of stone formation, magnesium and potassium, rose as well."

M K Terris 1, M M Issa, J R Tacker

Other sites suggest lower oxalate content which is why cranberries should be approached with real caution, and we've put a '3' in here.

Crawfish: 5

See fish for full explanation.

Crayfish: 5

See fish.

Cream cheeses: 5

Fine. See Cream below or Cheeses above.

Cream: 5

Fine. The University of Virginia Digestive Health Center notes:

Eat plenty of calcium-rich foods. Calcium binds to oxalate so that it isn't absorbed into your blood and cannot reach your kidneys. Dairy is free of oxalate and high in calcium, so it is an ideal choice. Choose skim, low fat, or full fat versions depending on your weight goals. If you are lactose intolerant, look for lactose free dairy such as Lactaid brand, or eat yogurt or kefir instead.

Cress: 1

Cress naturally contains extremely high amounts of oxalates. It's recommended that people who are at risk of experiencing urinary lithiasis absolutely reduce their intake of oxalate-rich foods like cress. They should not consume cress at all.

Cucumber: 5

Thought to be low in oxalate.

Cumin: 1

Cumin seeds are known for their higher oxalate content, but if you're seeking an alternative, online experts offer valuable insights into the world of spices.

They recommend less cumin and turmeric, and more garlic, lime, lemongrass, mint, and lots of lovely coconut which is thought to be low oxalate.

Curry: 3

Clearly not all curries are created equal. You want to check for ingredients and the level of spice and additives. This from PubMed:

Spices, such as cinnamon, cloves, cardamom, garlic, ginger, cumin, coriander and turmeric are used all over the world as flavouring and colouring ingredients in Indian foods. Previous studies have shown that spices contain variable amounts of total oxalates but there are few reports of soluble oxalate contents. In this study, the total, soluble and insoluble oxalate contents of ten different spices commonly used in Indian cuisine were measured. Total oxalate content ranged from 194 (nutmeg) to 4,014 (green cardamom) mg/100 g DM, while the soluble oxalate contents ranged from 41 (nutmeg) to 3,977 (green cardamom) mg/100 g DM. Overall, the percentage of soluble oxalate content of the spices ranged from 4.7 to 99.1% of the total oxalate content which suggests that some spices present no risk to people liable to kidney stone formation, while other spices can supply significant amounts of soluble oxalates and therefore should be used in moderation.

Dates: 2

High in oxalates with 24 mg per date according to the University of Chicago. They're also very high in sugar.

Dextrose: 5

See sugar.

Dill: 4

Low oxalate according to UPMC.

Dragon fruit: 1

Often known as white-fleshed pitahaya. High, 97.1 mg/100 g (source: Journal of Food Composition and Analysis).

Dried fruit: 3

Often high in oxalate. Watch out for pineapple and fig. Portion size can be a big issue. The University of Chicago notes.

Dried fruits have to be a worry because the water is taken out, so a 'portion' of dried fruit can be gigantic in oxalate content. Figs, pineapple and prunes are standouts. Just think: 1/2 cup of dried pineapple is 30 mg – not a lot of fruit for a lot of oxalate.

Elsewhere, canned pineapple are thought to be very high in oxalate, but canned cherries moderate, and canned pears and peaches little to no oxalate.

As previously seen, dates are oxalates with 24 mg per date according to the University of Chicago.

Dried meat: 5

Should be low in oxalates.

Dry-cured meats: 5

Should be low in oxalates.

Duck: 5

See meat.

Egg white: 5

Eggs are thought to be very low/no oxalate. However, moderation may be important if you are worried about kidney stones. The Harvard Health website notes;

Limit animal protein: Eating too much animal protein, such as red meat, poultry, eggs, and seafood, boosts the level of uric acid and could lead to kidney stones.4 Oct 2013

Egg yolk: 5

See comments above. Always buy organic and pasture-raised.

Elderflower cordial: 1

High. While elderberry fruits are a good source of minerals and antioxidants; the presence of oxalates and other anti-nutrients may limit their utilization.

Endive: 5

Thought to be low in oxalates.

Espresso: 5

See coffee.

Fennel: 1

High, 129 mg per 10 grams (source: Journal of Food Processing and Preservation).

Fenugreek: 2

According to a study, leafy vegetables such as curry, drumstick, shepu, fenugreek, coriander, radish, and onion stalks contain only insoluble oxalate, which ranges from 209.0 +/- 5.0 mg/100 g dry matter to 2,774.9 +/-18.4 mg/100 g dry matter (source: Journal of Food Processing and Preservation).

Feta cheese: 5

Thought to be low oxalate. See 'cheeses'.

Figs (fresh or dried): 3

See previous comments on figs and dried fruit. Dried figs are sometimes considered to have less than 5 mg of oxalate content per fig (source: University of Chicago), however portion size is important. May be a good alternative to dates that's high in fiber, potassium, iron, and calcium.

Fish: 5

Likely to be low oxalate. In addition, you may like to seek out fish with higher calcium levels; sardines with bones, whitebait, salmon and so on.

Flaxseed (linseed): 3

This is in the low- to moderate-oxalate group of foods, containing between 2 and 10 mg oxalate per 100 grams (source: UPMC).

Fructose (fruit sugar): 3

A study published in Pubmed explored reports that an increased fructose intake correspondingly increased the risk of forming kidney stones. It was postulated that fructose consumption increased urinary oxalate, a risk factor for calcium oxalate kidney stone disease. However, the subjects in the study did not demonstrate any changes in the excretions of oxalate, calcium, and uric acid.

Game (meat): 5

Low. However, eating large portions might increase the risk of kidney stones.

Garlic: 4

See broad-leaved garlic.

Ginger: 1

Contains an extensive amount of total oxalate (201-4014 mg/100 g) (source: Journal of Plant Foods for Human Nutrition).

Goat's milk: 5

See Milk.

Goji berry: 1

High.

Goose (organic, freshly cooked): 5

See meat.

Gooseberry, gooseberries: 1

Indian gooseberry is high oxalate.

Gouda cheese: 5

See cheese.

Grapefruit: 1

Very high. Thought to be one of the highest oxalate fruits unfortunately.

Grapes: 5

Thought to be low in oxalate. However, they are very high in sugar.

Green beans – see "beans"

Green peas: 5

Peas are thought to be low in oxalate with only 1mg of oxalate per half cup (source: St. Joseph's Healthcare Hamilton).

Green tea: 2

Wildly varies depending on the tea, and the investigative source.

Research shows that the amount of oxalate measured for black tea varies from 2.7 to 4.8 mg/240 mL (one cup) of tea infused for 1–5 min, whereas the amount of oxalate in green tea ranges from 2.08 to 34.94 mg/250 mL of tea (source: US National Library of Medicine).

However, the amount of oxalate in green tea depends on its origin, quality, preparation, and time of harvest, thus probably explaining why some studies report a higher oxalate concentration in black tea compared to green tea.

Guava: 1

High. Thought to change in oxalate content depending on ripeness.

Ham (dried, cured): 5

Low oxalate. However, eating large portions of meat is thought to potentially increase the risk of kidney stones.

Hazelnut: 1

High, best avoided. Nuts tend to be high in oxalates.

Hemp seeds (Cannabis sativa): 4

Nuts and seeds tend to be high in oxalates, but hemp seeds are thought to be a better choice. They contain just 3 mg oxalate per 2 tablespoons (source: https://www.thekidneydietitian.org/low-oxalate-nuts/).

Herbal tea: 3

Depends on the tea and the individual ingredients. Please look up the individual ingredients on list. Some teas, including black teas, are thought to accumulate a large amount of oxalates, resulting in a recommendation to eliminate black tea from your diet if you form oxalate stones (source: nature.com).

In a 2003 study, researchers from New Zealand discovered a 'tea hack'. They noted;

These studies show that consuming black tea on a daily basis will lead to a moderate intake of soluble oxalate each day, however the consumption of tea with milk on a regular basis will result in the absorption of very little oxalate from tea.

Honey: 5

See sweeteners.

Horseradish: 4

Some low oxalate experts recommend using this as a substitute for high-oxalate herbs and spices.

Particularly good with beef and seafood.

Juniper berries 5

Juniper berries are considered to be lithotriptic, which means that they help to dissolve and discharge urinary stones once they have formed. (source: Journal of Mazandaran University of Medical Sciences).

Kale: 5

Kale is thought to be low in oxalate, which makes it a good veggie choice.

Kefir: 5

Very low in oxalates. Cow's milk doesn't have oxalate so if Kefir is made from cow's milk, then it's a good choice. Note, Kefir can also be made from other sources.

Kelp: 3

Sometimes recommended as a nutrient to prevent kidney stones. This is because it's very high in calcium. Kelp is a type of seaweed, but oxalate content can vary from very high to very low depending on the specific kind of seaweed.

Kiwi: 1

Very high.

Kohlrabi: 5

Thought to be low in oxalate.

Lamb: 5

Low oxalate. See comments about meat.

Lamb's lettuce, corn salad: 5

See lettuce.

Lard: 5

Very low, less than 5 mg per 100 grams (source: University of Virginia).

Leek: 1

Leeks contain 89.0 mg of oxalate per 100 grams (source: UPMC).

Consume very moderately or avoid if you're on a low-oxalate diet.

Lemon: 3

A confusing one. Lemon is often considered to be low oxalate. However lemon peels are quite high in oxalate

- 83.0 mg per 100 grams - and lemon juice has just 1.0 mg per 100 g (source: UPMC).

Lentils: 4

Boiled lentils have low to moderate oxalate content.

Lettuce: 5

All kinds of lettuce are generally thought to be low in oxalates.

Lime: 3

Lime juice is thought to contain low amounts oxalates (between 2-5mg of oxalates per 100 grams according to various sources). It should be noted there is some divergence between lists.

Lime peels contain 110 mg per gram (source: UPMC). It's not often a person eats a lot of lime peel, but this would be something to be avoided.

Liquor: 4

See alcohol.

Liquorice: 1

One that is potentially on your 'culprits' list. Extremely high; licorice root had a total oxalate concentration of

3569 mg per 100 g. (source: Scientific Electronic Library of Brazil)

Lobster: 5

See notes under 'Fish'.

Loganberry: 1

Many nutritional benefits, but difficult to get reliable data on oxalate content. Test carefully.

Lychee: 5

Less than 2 mg of oxalate per 100 grams, (source: UPMC).

Macadamia: 1

Moderate to high, 10 – 25 mg per 100 grams (source: https://www.thekidneydietitian.org/low-oxalate-nuts/)

See *Nuts* for more information.

Malt extract: 1

High, best avoided

Malt: 1

High, best avoided.

Maltodextrin: 3

See sweeteners. Maltodextrin is often avoided by those looking to optimize a natural diet as it can be GMO and corn-derived.

Mandarin orange: 1

10 – 25 mg per 100 grams/ml, both for the fruit and the juice, this makes it moderately high in oxalates (source: UPMC) and high on list.

Mango: 2

10 - 25mg per 100 grams, moderate (source: UPMC). Consider to be moderate to high based on this and other food lists such as the Urinary Stones site.

Maple syrup: 3

Note previous comments about keeping sugar levels low for optimum health regardless of oxalate levels.

Margarine: 5

Low. However not always a great choice for general health because of the added preservatives.

Marrow: 5

Low.

Mascarpone cheese:

See other comments under Cheeses.

Mate tea: 2

Contains a moderate amount of oxalates.

Melon: 5

Cantaloupe, honeydew, and watermelon are all thought to be low in oxalate which is excellent news. A good fruit choice.

Milk: 5

Many on a low-oxalate diet seek out more calcium. The University of Virginia Digestive Health Center notes:

Eat plenty of calcium-rich foods. Calcium binds to oxalate so that it isn't absorbed into your blood and cannot reach your kidneys. Dairy is free of oxalate and high in calcium, so it is an ideal choice. Choose skim, low fat, or full fat versions depending on your weight goals. If you are lactose intolerant, look for lactosefree dairy such as Lactaid brand, or eat yogurt or kefir instead.

The respected Dr. Jockers says this about dairy products:

Dairy: Most food sources contain little to no oxalates. Examples include eggs, cheeses, yogurt, and plain milk (chocolate is a source of oxalates so stray from the chocolate milk).

Millet: 1

The grain is categorized as very high with over 15mg of oxalate per 100 g.

According to a study by the Cerials and Grains Association,

"The levels of total oxalate in raw cereals and millets varied greatly between 3.6 and 20.0 mg/100 g, and in cooked cereals and millets it ranged from 2.4 mg/100 g in rice to 13.4 mg/100 g in pearl millet... The levels of soluble oxalate in raw cereals and millets ranged from 1.9 to 9.1 mg/100 g."

Minced meat: 5

Low oxalate. However, eating large portions of meat is thought to potentially increase the risk of kidney stones.

Mint: 4

Mint tea is low in oxalates. Spearmint is moderate.

Morel: 2

Low.

Morello cherries: 4

Cherries are thought to be low in oxalate with around 2 mg per 100 grams (source: UPMC).

Canned Morello cherries are thought to be high in salicylates, a naturally occurring compound in plants.

Mozzarella cheese: 5

See other comments on soft cheeses.

Mulberry: 2

Calcium oxalate crystals are found in mulberry leaves.

Mungbeans (germinated, sprouting): 2

Moderate in oxalates, with around 8 mg of oxalate per half a cup (source: St. Joseph's Healthcare Hamilton).

Mushrooms, different types: 4

Low oxalate, but thoughts vary on how much, and the type of mushroom.

The University of Chicago suggests little or no oxalates in mushrooms.

Listed as 'Safe To Eat' on the Unusual Ingredients website.

Mustard and mustard seeds: 5

With just 0.1 - 2.9 mg per 100 g (source: Low Oxalate Diet - Mark O'Brien MD), all mustard is very low in oxalate.

Napa cabbage: 5

Cabbage is thought to be very low in oxalates along with similar veggies like endive and lettuce.

Nectarine: 5

It's thought to contain little to no oxalates.

Nettle tea: 3

Young leaves are not thought to have much oxalate. Do research before you consume nettles or nettle tea. Go slowly and carefully. The website KidneySchool notes:

If you make tea out of fresh nettle leaves, use small, young leaves. Older nettle leaves can contain oxalate, which can irritate the kidneys.

Research on PubMed suggests nettles may be good for kidney stones.

Urtica dioica or "Stinging Nettle", which belongs to the nettle genus of Urticaceae family, is used as tea in Austrian medicine [31,76]. It has shown a long history of beneficial therapeutic effects toward urinary ailments, specifically with the urinary tract and kidney stones. Its major bioactive phytochemicals include flavonoids, anthocyanins, and saponins [31]. These phytoconstituents provide the possibility of inhibition of calcium and oxalate deposition and crystals growth. Zhang H., Li N., Li K., Li P.

Nori seaweed: 4

Might help prevent kidney stones. Best consumed in moderation because it has very high iodine levels.

Nutmeg: 2

Thought to be low. Helen O'Connor, MS, RD lists this as containing 0-2mg of oxalates per serving.

Nuts: 1 (see individual nuts for more details)

Some say all nuts should be avoided on a Low-Oxalate diet. Check each individual nut. Almonds and Brazil nuts are thought to be particularly high. The website Kidney Dietitian notes;

Nuts & seeds are often taboo on a low oxalate, kidney stone friendly diet. This is probably because nuts and seeds are notorious for being high in oxalate. But, there are huge differences in oxalate between different nuts and seeds. If done correctly, nuts and seeds can be a part of a healthy low oxalate diet!

Oats: 5

Low. Making oats with milk instead of water is another way of increasing calcium.

Olive oil: 5

The site VP Foundation notes this is low oxalate, and so this book considers it to be an excellent healthy choice.

Olives: 2

The University of Chicago classifies them as very high with 18mg per 100 g. Best to avoid.

Onion: 5

Low oxalate.

Orange: 1

Generally high and best avoided. Peel especially so.

Oxalate content may depend on the size. A small orange (2⅜" diameter) is classified as moderate with 10 – 25 mg oxalates.

One teaspoon of raw orange peel contains 10 – 25 mg oxalates.

Orange juice is high in oxalates (source: St. Joseph's Healthcare Hamilton).

Oregano: 3

Low to moderate, dried oregano is listed as having 5 - 10 mg per 100 grams (source: Urinary Stones - Low Oxalate List).

Ostrich: 5

Low oxalate. However, eating large portions of meat is thought to potentially increase the risk of kidney stones.

Oyster: 5

Low, less than 5 mg per 100 grams (source: https://www.urinarystones.info/resources/Docs/Oxalate-content-of-food-2008.pdf)

Papaya: 5

Contains little to no oxalates.

Parsley: 2

Plenty of debate. Fresh parsley contains 5 – 10 mg per 100 grams, making it low to moderate in oxalates (source: https://www.urinarystones.info/resources/Docs/Oxalate-content-of-food-2008.pdf).

Others disagree. The Agriculture Handbook No. 8-11, Vegetables and Vegetable Products, 1984, lists Parsley as very high in oxalates.

The Heal With Food website notes about parsley and chives;

Like parsley, chives are generally only used in small amounts in cooking. Therefore, chives are not likely to contribute much oxalic acid to your diet, despite the fact they are among the most concentrated dietary sources of oxalates. A 100-serving of chives is estimated to provide 1480 milligrams of oxalates.

Parsnip: 2

High in oxalates, 15 mg per 100 g (University of Chicago).

Passion fruit: 5

Low.

Peach: 4

Thought to be low in oxalate and a good choice, although some disparity between lists.

Peanuts: 1

Thought to be very high in oxalates, like many nuts.

Pear: 4

Low however, note the high sugar content.

Peas (green): 5

Boiled peas are thought to be very low oxalate.

Pea Shoots (or pea sprouts): 3

Difficult to find consistent data, but eating moderate amounts of microgreens is less likely to cause the formation of kidney stones due to the higher citrate levels in microgreens which counterbalance the formation of calcium oxalate. Test carefully.

Peppermint tea: 5

Low; just 0.41 mg per cup (source: Pubmed, National Library of Medicine).

Pickled food: 1

Dill pickles are very low, pickled beets are extremely high.

Pineapple: 1

Low if fresh. Dried pineapple is very high with half a cup containing 30 mg (source: St. Joseph's Healthcare Hamilton).

Canned pineapple also to be avoided.

Pistachio: 1

14mgper1/4cup(source:https://www.thekidneydietitian.org/low-oxalate-nuts/#Pistachios). And who only eats 1/4 cup of pistachios at once? 49mg per 100g according to the PainSpy Low Oxalate Diet Foods List.

Plum: 5

Thought to contain little to no oxalates.

Pomegranate: 1

High.

Poppy seeds: 1

High.

Pork: 5

See meat.

Potato: 1

Dr. Jockers lists potato in his High-Oxalate Foods list. A medium baked potato has 50 milligrams of oxalates per 100g according to the Pain Spy Low Oxalate Foods List, but other sources say you can lower this by getting rid of the skin.

(This is also considered to be the same with pears which are lower oxalate when you take the skin off). That's where many of the oxalates are.

On the other hand, the skin contains fiber, vitamin C, B vitamins, and other healthy nutrients (source: St. Joseph's Healthcare Hamilton).

Poultry meat: 5

Low oxalate. However, eating large portions of meat is thought to potentially increase the risk of kidney stones. Non-organic would also potentially get a lower score on the general health front.

Prawn: 5

Low, like most seafood.

Processed cheese:

See cheese.

Prune: 2

Dried prune is very high in oxalates. Prune juice is thought to be moderate in oxalates. Proceed with caution.

Pulses: 1

Pulses include peas, lentils, fava beans, chickpeas, and common beans. These vary widely so check individually.

According to PubMed, pulses can be very high in oxalates. Oxalate content varies, ranging from 244.7-294.0 mg/100 g in peas, 168.6-289.1 mg/100 g in lentils, 241.5-291.4 mg/100 g in fava beans, 92.2-214.0 mg/100 g in chickpeas and 98.86-117.0 mg/100 g in common beans. Approximately 24-72% of total oxalate appeared to be soluble in all investigated pulses.

It notes;

Soaking the seeds in distilled water significantly decreased the contents of total oxalate (17.40-51.89%) and soluble oxalate (26.66-56.29%).

Pumpkin seed oil: 3

See Pumpkin seeds below.

Pumpkin seeds: 3

Considerable debate. Consume in small portions. The website Kidney Dietitian notes:

Pumpkin seeds* (or "pepitas") are more than a treat in the fall! You can find pumpkin seeds year round. Add them to *salads, oatmeal, yogurt or make your own low oxalate trail mix! 5 mg oxalate per 1/4 cup.*

Pumpkin: 4

Canned pumpkins are thought to have very low content and raw pumpkins negligible. Pumpkin seeds are different - see above.

Quinoa: 1

Thought to be high in oxalates. Approach with caution.

Rabbit: 5

Low oxalate. However, eating large portions of meat is thought to potentially increase the risk of kidney stones.

Raclette cheese: 5

See cheeses. Thought to be low oxalate.

Radish: 5

White radish is considered to be low in oxalates, red radish is considered to be very low.

Raisins: 4

Low but not negligible.

Rapeseed oil (called canola oil in US): 5

The site The VP Foundation notes all vegetable oils, including olive, canola, safflower, and soy and margarine are low oxalate.

Regardless of oxalates, this book considers it one to avoid this as many believe at times rapeseed oil can cause inflammation. But you might tolerate it well.

Raspberry: 1

Considered to be high in oxalates. One 100 g size contains around 48 mg of oxalates according to the University of Chicago. However the Pain Spy Low Oxalate Foods List considers there to be 55mg of oxalates in black raspberries and 15mg in red raspberries.

Raspberries are one of the lowest sugar fruits.

Raw milk: 5

Raw milk is thought to be very low in oxalates. The University of Virginia Digestive Health Center advises:

Eat plenty of calcium-rich foods. Calcium binds to oxalate so that it isn't absorbed into your blood and cannot reach your kidneys. Dairy is free of oxalate and high in calcium, so it is an ideal choice. Choose skim, low fat, or full fat versions depending on your weight goals. If you are lactose intolerant, look for lactose-free dairy such as Lactaid brand, or eat yogurt or kefir instead.

Red cabbage: 5

Thought to be low in oxalates.

Red wine vinegar: 5

Thought to be low in oxalate. See other vinegars for more details.

Redcurrants: 1

Winchester Hospital lists them as high and best avoided.

Rhubarb: 1

Thought to contain massive amounts of oxalates. On very close inspection of the food lists, estimated between 541 mg and 800 mg per 100 grams, making it one of the oxalate-loaded foods around.

This makes it one of the highest oxalate foods in this book.

All of which means you'll sadly have to avoid rhubarb crumble on a low oxalate diet, but you could replace with apple crumble.

Rice: 3

Varies considerably depending on the rice.

White rice tends to be very low oxalate, but brown rice is thought to be moderate. Winchester Hospital qualifies wild rice as low oxalate. Black rice is high in oxalates.

Rice cakes: 4

See Rice.

Rice milk: 3

See Rice. Watch out for added ingredients in rice milks. As a rule of thumb, the fewer ingredients, the better.

Rice noodles: 3

See Rice.

Ricotta cheese: 5

Cheeses are generally considered low in oxalate.

Rooibos tea: 5

Just 0.55-1.06 mg of oxalate per cup based on steep time (source: Pubmed, National Library of Medicine). The site lowoxalateinfo.com notes:

Rooibos is the first low oxalate tea I have found that both tastes great and is full-bodied enough to enjoy hot with cream.

Roquefort cheese: 5

Cheeses are thought to be low oxalate.

Rosemary: 5

Low in oxalates.

Rum: 4

See alcohol.

Rye: 1

Rye flour is moderate to high in oxalates. The unprocessed grain itself is very high with at least 15.0 mg per 100 g (source: Urinary Stones Food List).

Sage: 5

UPMC lists as low oxalate.

Salami: 5

Low oxalate. However, eating large portions of meat is thought to potentially increase the risk of kidney stones. Cured meats are generally considered bad for your health.

Salmon: 5

Good news, salmon is considered to have little or no oxalates, like most fish.

Sauerkraut: 4

Low, you can have it in any quantity, although you should still combine it with calcium.

Sausages of all kinds: 5

See meat.

Savoy cabbage: 5

Thought to be low in oxalates.

Schnapps: 4

See 'Alcohol'.

Seafood: 5

Low.

Seaweed: 4

Varies. Some kinds are thought to prevent the formation of calcium oxalate kidney stones. Research published in the Journal of Functional Foods shows that sulphated polysaccharides (SPSs) from various seaweeds possess broad spectrum therapeutic and biomedical properties that are known to play a significant inhibitory role in these stones.

Sesame: 1

15.0 mg & up per 100 g, very high oxalate content (source: Urinary Stones - The Oxalate Content Of Food).

Sheep's milk, sheep milk: 5

See milk.

Shellfish: 5

Low, as per seafood in general

Shrimp: 5

Low, as per seafood in general

Smoked fish: 5

See fish.

Smoked meat: 5

Low oxalate. However, eating large portions of meat is thought to potentially increase the risk of kidney stones.

Snow peas – see "green peas"

Soft cheese: 5

See comments under 'Cheese'.

Sour cream: 5

Sour cream is a good choice for people on a low oxalate diet. The University of Virginia Digestive Health Center advises:

Eat plenty of calcium-rich foods. Calcium binds to oxalate so that it isn't absorbed into your blood and cannot reach your kidneys. Dairy is free of oxalate and high in calcium, so it is an ideal choice. Choose skim, low fat, or full fat versions depending on your weight goals. If you are lactose intolerant, look for lactose-free dairy such as Lactaid brand, or eat yogurt or kefir instead.

Soy (soy beans, soy flour): 1

Potentially high in oxalate depending on the soy product. Soy flour is thought to be particularly high in oxalates. Approach each individual soy product carefully.

Website WebMD notes;

Products made from soybeans are excellent sources of protein and other nutrients, especially for people on a plant-based diet. However, they are also high in oxalates.

Soy sauce: 2

Approach all soy products with caution. The good news is that soy sauce may be lower in oxalate than other soy products, such as soy flour.

Sparkling wine: 4

See alcohol.

Spelt: 3

Difficult to find reliable information. Test carefully. Fun fact: Spelt was one of the first grains to be used to make bread.

Spinach: 1

Very high in oxalates. One of the highest oxalate foods. The website WebMD notes;

Leafy greens like spinach contain many vitamins and minerals, but they're also high in oxalates. A half-cup of cooked spinach contains 755 milligrams.

If you must eat spinach, it's thought cooking it *may* reduce the oxalate levels, but only to around 650 mg per half cup.

Spirits: 4

See alcohol.

Squashes: 3

Squash seeds are thought to be low, or low to moderate, 5-10mg per 100 grams. Cooked summer squash and winter squash are moderate, 10 - 25mg per 100 grams (source: Urinary Stones - The Oxalate Content Of Food).

Stevia: 1

Plenty of disagreement online about stevia (as there is about many foods in this book). Website WebMD puts stevia in their high oxalate food category. Chemical stevia has no oxalate.

Stinging nettle: 3

Stinging nettle can help prevent and possibly dissolve kidney stones and gout because its extract decreases elevated levels of calcium, oxalate, and creatinine in urine. One study showed it significantly limited the amount of calcium and oxalate and calcium oxalate crystals in the kidneys of test rats (source: Pubmed).

Strawberry: 5

Thought to be low in oxalates. Winchester Hospital lists strawberries in their Foods safe-to-eat category.

Sugar: 5

Sugar is thought to be low oxalate, but is not good for those with certain health issues. Look into alternatives. The University of Chicago writes on its Kidney Stones site:

Just one sugared drink raises your urine calcium within 30 minutes and keeps it up for at least 2 hours more. At the same time, it lowers your urine volume. If you have hypercalciuria – a majority of stone formers have it – the effect is larger because you start higher, and your urine volume will fall more. So with every sugary treat, risk of making stones increases for hours.

Sunflower oil: 4

Low oxalate, however can cause inflammation. Test carefully.

Sunflower seeds: 3

Some say low, just 3 mg oxalate per 1/4 cup (source: https://www.thekidneydietitian.org/low-oxalate-nuts/)

However other sources like Kidney Cop list these as "high oxalate foods that you should avoid or minimize with calcium oxalate stones."

There is enough debate that this has been revisited in the second edition of this book.

Sweetcorn: 3

Moderate.

Sweet potato: 1

Considered to be very high in oxalates, with some estimating 28 mg per 100 g (source: Scientific Electronic Library Online of Brazil).

Dr. Jockers says this on his excellent website.

I teach my clients to minimize their consumption of spinach, beets, grains, nuts, sweet potatoes and chocolate for 3 months

Tea, black: 1

Some teas including black teas are thought to accumulate a large amount of oxalates, resulting in a recommendation to eliminate black tea from your diet if you tend to form oxalate stones (source: nature.com).

In a 2003 study, researchers from New Zealand discovered a 'tea hack'. They noted;

These studies show that consuming black tea on a daily basis will lead to a moderate intake of soluble oxalate each day, however the consumption of tea with milk on a regular basis will result in the absorption of very little oxalate from tea.

Thyme: 4

Dried thyme is thought to contain low to moderate levels of oxalate.

Tomato: 1

Moderate to high.

Trout: 5

See fish.

Tuna: 5

Like most fish, it's low in oxalates, but tends to have a high heavy metal content.

Turkey: 5

Meat has little to no oxalates.

Turmeric: 1

Many experts consider this to be the highest oxalate-containing spice.

Turnip: 1

Very high in oxalates, 30 mg per 100 g (University of Chicago).

Vanilla: 1

Lists vary. Challenging to get consistent information therefore scored a 1. Includes vanilla, vanilla extract, vanilla pod, vanilla powder, vanilla sugar.

Venison: 5

See meat.

Vinegar: balsamic: 5

5-10 mg per 100 g, low (source: Urinary Stones - The Oxalate Content Of Food).

Vinegar: distilled white vinegar: 5

Very low, less than 5 mg per 100 g (source: Urinary Stones - The Oxalate Content Of Food).

Walnut: 1

Thought to be very high in oxalates. Some say all nuts should be avoided on a Low-Oxalate diet.

Watercress: 1

High, best avoided. See cress for more info.

Watermelon: 5

See melon.

Wheat: 1

Some debate. Dr. Jockers lists in his High-Oxalate Food List category.

In addition, many people observe giving up gluten does help their overall wellness levels so this is something you may want to consider.

Wheat germ: 1

A study in Pubmed showed high total oxalate content (>50 mg/100 g) in the whole grain wheat species Triticum durum (76.6 mg/100 g), Triticum sativum (71.2 mg/100 g), and Triticum aestivum (53.3 mg/100 g).

White button mushroom: 4

See mushrooms.

Wild rice: 3

See comments on 'Rice'. Rice varies considerably by type.

Wine: 4

See alcohol.

Yam: 1

Very high in oxalates, 40 mg per 100 g (University of Chicago).

Yeast: 2

Yeast as a baking ingredient has been found moderately high in oxalate content.

Yogurt/Yoghurt: 5

Very low in oxalate, although often high in sugar. The University of Virginia Digestive Health Center advises:

Eat plenty of calcium-rich foods. Calcium binds to oxalate so that it isn't absorbed into your blood and cannot reach your kidneys. Dairy is free of oxalate and high in calcium, so it is an ideal choice. Choose skim, low fat, or full fat versions depending on your weight goals. If you are lactose intolerant, look for lactose-free dairy such as Lactaid brand, or eat yogurt or kefir instead.

Zucchini: 5

Thought to be low oxalate by most sources. Also known as courgette. Includes marrow.

Easy Low-Oxalate Shopping List

Acerola

Alcohol

Algae

Anchovies

Apple

Apple cider vinegar

Apricot

Banana

Barley

Basil

Beef

Beer

Bison

Bivalves (mussels, oyster, clams, scallops)

Bok choi

Boysenberry

Brandy

Broad-leaved garlic

Butter

Cabbage

Cauliflower

Cep mushrooms

Chamomile and chamomile tea

Champagne

Cherry

Cheddar cheese

Cheese made from unpasteurized "raw" milk

Cheeses

Chicken

Chicory

Chives

Cilantro (Coriander)

Coconut and coconut derivatives

Cress

Coffee

Corn salad, lamb's lettuce

Cornflakes

Courgette

Crab

Crawfish

Crayfish

Cream cheeses

Cream

Cucumber

Dextrose

Dill

Dried meat

Dry-cured meats

Duck

Egg white

Egg yolk

Endive

Espresso

Feta cheese

Fish

Game (meat)

Garlic

Goat's milk

Goose (organic, freshly cooked)

Gouda cheese

Grapes

Green peas

Ham (dried, cured)

Hemp seeds (Cannabis sativa)

Honey

Horseradish

Juniper berries

Kale

Kefir

Kohlrabi

Lamb

Lamb's lettuce, corn salad

Lard

Lentils

Lobster

Lychee

Lettuce

Liquor

Margarine

Marrow

Mascarpone cheese

Melon

Milk

Minced meat

Mint

Morello cherries

Mozzarella cheese

Mushrooms, different types

Mustard and mustard seeds

Napa cabbage

Nectarine

Nori seaweed

Oats

Olive oil

Onion

Ostrich

Oyster

Peach

Pear

Peas (green)

Papaya

Passion fruit

Peppermint tea

Plum

Pork

Poultry meat

Prawn

Processed cheese

Pumpkin

Rabbit

Raclette cheese

Radish

Raisins

Rice cakes

Rapeseed oil (called canola oil in US)

Raw milk

Red cabbage

Ricotta cheese

Rooibos tea

Roquefort cheese

Rosemary

Rum

Sage

Salami

Salmon

Sauerkraut

Sausages of all kinds

Savoy cabbage

Schnapps

Seafood

Seaweed

Sheep's milk, sheep milk

Shellfish

Shrimp

Smoked fish

Smoked meat

Snow peas

Soft cheese

Sour cream

Sparkling wine

Spirits

Strawberry

Sugar

Thyme

Trout

Tuna

Turkey

Venison

Watermelon

White Rice

White button mushroom

Yogurt/Yoghurt

Zucchini/Courgette

At a glance food lists for the low-oxalate diet.

Pantry Staples: (as always check individual ingredients and tolerance levels carefully before adding to diet)

- Olive oil
- Apple cider vinegar
- Honey
- Sugar
- White Rice
- Coffee
- Cornflakes
- Corn flour

Go-to Simple Dinner Ingredients:

- Chicken
- Beef
- Bison
- Cabbage
- Cauliflower
- Cucumber

- Lettuce
- Zucchini/Courgette
- Mushroom varieties
- Garlic

Favorite Fruits

- Apple
- Banana
- Pear
- Grapes
- Plum
- Cherry
- Watermelon
- Melon
- Nectarine

In a Hurry:

- Canned tuna
- Eggs
- Butter
- Cheeses (check list for individual cheeses)
- Cornflakes
- Rice cakes
- Ham
- Yogurt

- Frozen peas
- Cucumber

Fancy Dinner:

- Lobster
- Crab
- Duck
- Game (meat)
- Trout
- Brandy (for cooking)
- Champagne
- Smoked fish
- Roquefort cheese
- Gouda cheese

Made in the USA
Las Vegas, NV
04 June 2024